Stick It in Your Ear

Deano Kinsey

DEDICATION

This book is dedicated to my father. It was he who originally suggested that I take a look at the hearing aid field, during an extended period of unemployment in the early 2000's. Amidst many other family suggestions, my father with the Alzheimer's, had made a suggestion that would change both our lives. I ended up giving dad *and* mom better hearing in the sunset of his life. My dad gave me a second career, where I now help others every day.

CONTENTS

1 There May Be a Problem Here   Pg 1

2 I Can Hear Just Fine   Pg 7

3 Getting Unstuck   Pg 13

4 How We Hear   Pg 22

5 Ignoring the Problem and the Consequences   Pg 30

6 The Hearing Test   Pg 34

7 Buying Hearing Aids   Pg 47

8 Life with Hearing Aids   Pg 65

9 Hearing Aids Don't Fix Everything   Pg 75

10 Conclusion   Pg 81

ACKNOWLEDGMENTS

The author would like to acknowledge the influences of my mentors, Eric Stratton and Geoff Calkins. The best skills are passed on to me by these experts who work tirelessly to improve lives every day. These men were instrumental in my training, and I am forever grateful to them. Cover art by Travis Kinsey.

Chapter 1

There May Be a Problem Here

Hearing loss usually occurs over a long period of time; it develops very slowly. It can happen so slowly that the sufferer doesn't really notice the effects. In fact, it is usually those around the hearing loss sufferer that notice it first.

It starts with the huhs and the whats and continues with more and more requests to repeat information. Then simple misunderstandings begin to happen, like giving the answer to the wrong question. This happens slowly over time, and the person who is around the sufferer the most can begin to turn into the human hearing aid.

There are literally millions of people with varying degrees of hearing loss who cope with its effects every day. Those around them cope with it every day too. The average person waits five to ten years to seek help after noticing a problem. So what happens is that you have a problem that can build up over time. Many times, by the time the sufferer seeks help, the significant other in their life is pretty much at their wits end.

One of the coping mechanisms for dealing with a hearing loss is to simply give up. That is, becoming gradually more and more isolated from others. Sufferers will stop asking for so many repeats because the people who are repeating to them have started giving negative feedback, expressing their dismay at the sufferer. Often times in a multiple person conversation, the hearing loss sufferer will sit there, trying to listen but only catch part of what is being said. They really are not getting all of the information, so they fake it.

Another thing that really starts to isolate hearing loss sufferers is embarrassment and shame. If you are embarrassed about not being able to hear, and you know others are aware of this, you begin to exclude those activities that reveal your hearing loss to others. Quitting clubs and meetings due to embarrassment over a hearing loss is very common. This is also the beginning of the slippery slope of increased isolation.

I hear stories every day about that what Dr. Phil calls that 'pivotal moment' which moves the person to get a hearing evaluation, that uncomfortable moment when someone becomes 'unstuck' and decides to at least have their hearing evaluated. I actually cut right to the chase, in the first few minutes of the hearing evaluation intake. I look the person sitting in the chair in the eye, and I ask them: "How did you end up in my chair?" Then I listen.

Many, many people land in my chair because of negative feedback from others around them. Essentially what is happening is that others are tired of having the patient's hearing problem translate into a problem for them. The constant repeats, clarifications, misunderstandings, loud TV and radio volumes, often prompt the sufferer to seek help.

I observed both types of responses to hearing loss in my own family; with both of my grandparents. My grandma has worn hearing aids for many years now. Grandpa however, has had a hearing problem for a time now, and wouldn't even get a hearing test. He refused to even acknowledge that he may even have a problem. So you can imagine my grandparent's home life. Grandma wears hearing aids, and grandpa has an obvious hearing problem, and won't do anything about it. The difference in what each of them need for sound stimulus is great. Grandma can hear TV at volume 10, but grandpa can't hear it unless it is at volume 25.

So I was going to throw a big party for my fiftieth birthday. As things turned out, Grandpa was going to be the first to arrive coming in about five days early. I relished the thought of some quality time with him, in the calm before what was sure to be the party storm. With a house full of family, and with 50-60 guests at a rented winery, it was going to be a big deal.

Well, three days before Grandpa's arrival, my new, big screen TV quit working. Great. So, I ended up renting one while mine was being replaced. Grandpa had mentioned that he was looking forward to seeing some sports on my fancy TV, so I couldn't let him down.

Grandma has worn hearing aids for years now, but Grandpa refused to even be tested. We knew that he had some sort of hearing problems, but he would have nothing to do with any help. Repeats for him, talking louder for him, loud TV, the whole array of coping mechanisms were in play for him to avoid the problem.

It must have been nearly midnight on the evening before the mass of family house guests arrived, and I was beat. Grandpa had been having a great time thus far. I had no trouble with the loud TV and our challenging communications all week, but apparently my patience was waning.

I was trying to get to sleep, with a million things on my mind with the party just two days away now. Grandpa has the TV up loud again, and it is golf. That's right, golf at 90 decibels at midnight. It was a bad combination, and I snapped. I jumped out of bed and threw on a house coat and flew out of my bedroom door. From the top of the stairs, I could see Grandpa on the couch downstairs. I yelled down to him: "Turn that thing down! I feel like a prisoner in my own home!" He had this scared look on his face, and went ahead and turned the TV off altogether, and we retired for the evening.

Nothing was said the next morning, but two days later, Grandpa asked me to test his hearing. For grandpa, this was his 'pivotal moment'. And this is just one example of how people end up in the hearing aid office chair. He has since become a successful hearing aid wearer.

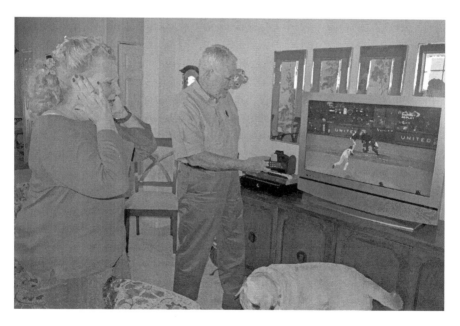

"Turn that thing down!"

Others land in my chair because they readily acknowledge that they have a hearing problem, or suspect so, and are actively engaged in testing and hopefully finding some help. In many cases, getting a hearing test and perhaps considering hearing aids is better than continuing to endure disdain from friends and family.

Here are some other examples of how people end up in the hearing aid office chair:

- The schoolteacher: "I struggle to hear student's voices; especially when I am writing on the board and the students speaking to me are at the back of the classroom."

- The executive: "In meetings, I have a very difficult time hearing some of the people at the table."

- The doctor: "It is vital that I hear what my patients are telling me and sometimes I worry about what they must think when I ask them to repeat."

- The construction worker: "My guys have really started to give me a hard time when I can't understand them the first time."

- The salesman: "People start to get irritated with me if I ask them to repeat too many times; it is embarrassing."

- A nurse: "Some of my sickest patients can't speak very loudly, and I feel so bad when I have to ask them several times what they said."

- The retiree: "I can't always hear the number that is called, and I wonder how many times I have missed a bingo."

- The wife: "My bridge partner has gotten pretty upset with me a few times for my silly responses to comments."

I tell people in my office that I have the one thing in the entire store that nobody wants, but many people need. I also tell people that I can improve their home life. Some people look at me when I say this, as if they are thinking that I am like some slick car salesman, spewing some lofty outcome that I couldn't possibly ever deliver on. These doubters are the last to understand the very real improvement a properly fitted hearing aid can provide.

Summary

✓ Hearing loss usually comes on very slowly.

✓ Many people who have hearing loss don't know it, can't accept it or won't do anything about it.

✓ The average person waits five to ten years to get help.

✓ There are millions of people with varying degrees of hearing loss.

✓ People with hearing loss can gradually become more and more isolated from others.

✓ Embarrassment and shame can accompany hearing loss.

Chapter 2

I Can Hear Just Fine

Since a hearing problem usually develops over a long period of time, it really does tend to sneak up on people. And, the classic refrain from many of those people is that their hearing is fine. They are either unable to notice, or unwilling to accept, that they have trouble hearing.

It is no secret to those people around or living with someone who has a hearing problem. Day in and day out, week in and week out, life can be more challenging for everyone who has to communicate with a person who can't hear very well. In many homes, the person with the hearing problem causes stress and frustration amongst those that are trying to communicate with him or her. He or she will most likely have added stress and frustration also as they try to understand and be understood.

Sitting in their kitchen, a man and woman are chatting. The woman has suspected that she has had a hearing problem for some time. They have had a few misunderstandings in the past. So one afternoon, the man says to her, "Hey baby, how would you like a hot spicy peanut?" She looks at him and blurts out "How dare you talk to me like that!" The man was startled and puzzled. It turns out that initially she heard something different; she thought he was talking about a male body part.

She was in the chair the next day.

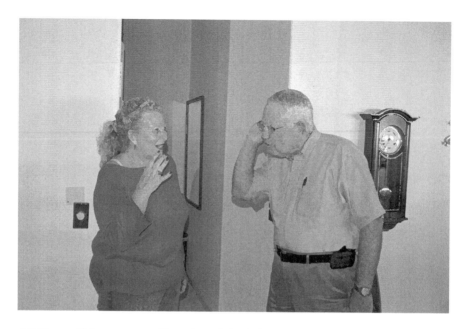

"What did you say (for the third time)?"

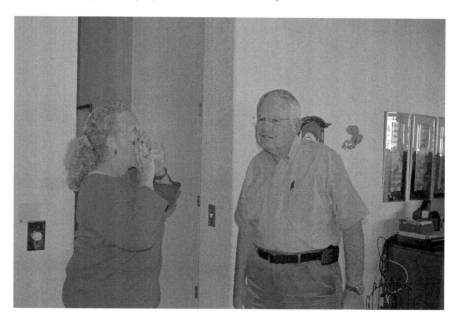

"I SAID…..!"

Many times, all of the participants or players in these settings end up doing a familiar dance with the person who has the hearing problem. You say this, he says huh? You say it louder, he says huh? You get irritated and shout it out, and he gets irritated that you are yelling at him. And there you go again: that familiar back and forth dance, with each player playing their role in a painfully consistent and frustrating fashion. Sound familiar?

Then there is the "heard it wrong" dance. You say a certain word in a sentence that isn't heard correctly, and then the meaning of the whole sentence changes for the listener. They come back with something totally different than your intended meaning, thinking that they heard it correctly. You now find yourselves trying to get to the meaning of a sentence or idea. It takes twice as long to get something across, which takes a toll if it continues on a long term basis. Sound familiar?

So this gentleman goes to his doctor and tells the doctor that he is concerned about his wife's hearing. The doctor gives the man some instructions to go home with, so he can casually test his wife's hearing.

The gentleman heads home, and the wife is in the yard watering. With her back to him and about 30 feet away, he asks his wife 'what is for dinner? He hears no answer. He moves up five feet, and asks the question again. And again, there is no answer. So he moves up another five feet and asks the question again, and no answer again.

One more time, he moves up five feet and asks the question, and once again, no answer. Okay he thinks, at fifteen feet, she should hear me, and he asks the question. Again, he hears no response. His suspicions are now seeming to be true, when he moves within five feet, and asks his wife 'what is for dinner? He finally hears her answer back: 'For the sixth time, we are having chicken for dinner!'

There are a million varieties of coping mechanisms on the part of the person with the hearing problem. Equally, there are many coping mechanisms on the part of those people trying to communicate with that person with hearing trouble. Some of these coping strategies are kind and helpful. In other cases, these coping strategies can turn into negative feedback and anger towards the person with challenged hearing.

The large majority of men and women who end up in my chair are there because of negative feedback from others. And almost always, that comes from the spouse or adult children, and this makes sense. Those closest to the hearing challenged are the most affected. They usually get sick and tired of coping with the challenge of communicating, over and over and over.

The average time a person waits to get help with their hearing problem is five to ten years *from the time they first notice a problem.* That's right, up to ten years and perhaps longer. This is a considerable chunk of time for family, friends and loved ones to cope with a problem of someone else's.

This passage of time coping with the same problem, over and over, can lead to a buildup of animosity and anger. This can strain what otherwise may be a healthy and happy relationship.

In summary, people who time after time say that they can hear just fine, are only going to be able to buy so much time before the negativity, anger or embarrassment become bothersome enough to spur a person to action.

There are a whole host of reasons why people resist taking steps to solve their hearing problems. Here are a few:

- Denial

- Selfishness

- Pride

- Shame

- Anger

- Cost

- Perception

- Falsehoods

- Stigma

These will be explored in depth later.

It turns out that it can take quite a while to learn or accept that you may have a hearing problem. It can take even longer to seek out help. I tell everyone that I have the one healthcare device that is way better than it used to be and can really help them a lot.

Summary

- ✓ It can take a long time to lose one's hearing.

- ✓ It can take five to ten years *after noticing* a problem, before action is taken.

- ✓ Friends and family are usually the ones to spur action.

- ✓ There are those 'dances' that we all do to get around the issue.

- ✓ Negative feedback is the usual reason for seeking hearing help.

Chapter 3

Getting Unstuck

Okay, so there may be a problem, you may or may not hear just fine. By now you, yourself or others suspect that you have a hearing problem. Things are happening frequently now that really seem to point in the direction of some hearing issues.

It might be the incessant *huhs?* and *whats?*. It might be that old 'you said this, I heard that' dance. It might be the loud TV volume. If you have trouble hearing, there will be clues. You have to decide if you are going to pay attention to those clues, or ignore them. Some people simply ignore the clues. Others don't care. Yet others deny that a problem exists: it has to be others mumbling; they don't speak clearly; etc.

In a perfect world, a person would become quickly aware of a hearing problem, or any other health problem for that matter. He or she, would learn of a problem, promptly seek help for the problem, and have it addressed by a healthcare professional. We as people unfortunately, are not perfect. We are skeptical. We ignore. We deny. We avoid. We make assumptions. Seldom are we so inspired as to have every facet of our lives nailed down and in control at every moment.

Then, as we get older, we begin to lose things that we once took for granted. After age forty, our eyesight can become less clear. We may have less hair. We may no longer be skinny. We may have less get up and go. We may not hear like we used to.

All of these things remind us that we are not young any more. And for many, the reminder that carries by far the biggest impact? Oh god, I may need hearing aids.

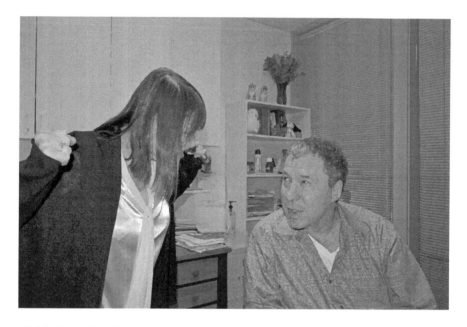

"Oh My God! Repeat, repeat, repeat; you are driving me crazy!"

There are a whole host of reasons why people resist taking steps to solve their hearing problems. Here are a few:

Denial- The person cannot accept that there may be a problem.

Selfishness - There is a problem, and they don't care. It's other people's problem.

Pride - The person isn't able to cope with something 'only others need'.

Shame - There is a reluctance to be seen wearing a hearing instrument.

Anger – The 'why me' reaction to poor hearing.

Stigma - This signifies that I am old and everyone will find out.

Perception - Hearing problems are 'only for the elderly'.

Falsehoods - Everyone who wears hearing aids is unhappy with them.

Cost - The high price keeps help out of financial reach.

Getting Unstuck

I see all flavors of people in my office who have a hearing loss. Some of them are eager for the help; they wear their hearing aids every day and love the help that they receive. They shower me with glowing praise, they hug me, and they try to give me gifts. They tell their friends, and some of them come in for help too.

Then of course, there are some people who are kicking and screaming and don't want anything to do with hearing aids. They are in my office against their will and want to make sure I know it. These people most likely will be revealed to have a hearing loss, but really don't want any help. For one or more of the reasons as mentioned before, they are unwilling to entertain the idea of getting help.

There are no quick and easy answers for getting anyone to get tested or to start wearing hearing aids. It can be useful to arm yourself with information, in case you may be forced into a position of 'coaxing' someone to get help.

First of all, consider some of the problems in the household that poor hearing can affect:

- Loud television.
- Constant stress of communication.
- Anger from you or the sufferer.
- Yelling matches between household members.
- Misunderstandings with negative consequences.
- Not hearing alarms or warning beeps or tones (safety).

Now consider some of the problems outside the home:

- Understanding and following directions.
- Listening to service providers.
- Interacting with waiters and clerks, etc.
- Interacting with people in public.
- Obeying warning sounds (safety).

In view of some of the issues both in and out of the home, it is no wonder that at some point, someone has to decide to do something. How long do normal-hearing people put up with these things? How long is it before something happens that could be a safety issue? These are the things that many people wrestle with as they attempt to find help for a hearing problem.

There are three main categories of people who buy hearing aids:

- They know that they have a problem and they embrace the help.
- They have a problem and don't embrace the help until it proves to be a positive outcome.
- They have a problem and they don't accept or don't want a solution.

The easiest people to help get unstuck are those who accept that they have a problem. A little prodding and a few embarrassing moments easily illustrate to these people that they need to seek help for their hearing problem. And generally, if they can get a decent price and a good fit, they will wear their hearing aids and reap the rewards of being back in the conversation.

The middle group of those people who don't readily accept that they have a problem can be a challenge. This group either can't or won't accept that they have a problem. This usually means that someone, like a spouse or someone close to them has had enough and forces action. This person has had hearing issues for a while, and now they are forced into a hearing test and most likely purchasing and wearing hearing aids. If they get a decent price, and if they get a good fit, they may wear them. Some prodding on a daily basis in the beginning may be needed to coax them into regular use.

What happens with this category of people is that as they wear their hearing aids more and more, they begin to develop a positive addiction to hearing better again. It doesn't really take a whole lot of effort to get them to wear their hearing aids once they hear for themselves. Being included again, understanding and being a part of conversation again and hearing things that were difficult before will convince this category of people. It is an amazing turn around. Time and again, the person who came in kicking and screaming against hearing aids in the beginning has become a convert. They now depend on hearing aids and can't live without them.

There have been people in my office who were close to being rude they were so against even being in my office. Over the space of a few weeks or months, they come around and end up embracing better hearing and then, one hearing aid may break. I tell them that it needs to stay in the office and get fixed. Then the funniest thing happens: The person, who was once kicking and screaming against hearing aids, will now sit there and exclaim "You can't take that away from me, I NEED it to hear with!" It is an amazing turn-around that happens quite a bit actually.

The last category of people is the most difficult. They can't or won't accept that they have a hearing problem, and they can't or won't accept any help. No matter what approach is taken, there is no movement, no bending, no hearing test and simply no way that they will consider hearing aids. This group of people requires the most prodding and sometimes outright threatening to get them to move. And sadly, many times if they can be convinced to try hearing aids they will either return them, or simply not wear them.

It is important to at least try to help the seemingly un-helpable. Even a small percentage of this group ends up 'seeing the light' so to speak.

Here are few tips on getting people unstuck:

- If you love me, you will get help for your problem.
- It is a safety issue, you keep missing important things like cars and the beeper on the baby monitor.
- Your buddy so and so got hearing aids and look what a difference they have made for him.
- They are cheaper than a divorce!
- Our marriage is suffering more and more because of your hearing problem.
- They are not the big, clunky things that they used to be.
- Our friends will think more of you, not less of you if you can hear well.
- The grandkids don't understand why you can't understand them; they are giving up trying to talk to you.
- Peer pressure in small, consistent doses.

Peer pressure ends up usually being the most effective way to get people unstuck. Have their friends and loved ones give them negative feedback, over and over. Usually, people will respond to peer pressure way faster than simply having the wife or husband nagging for years. Get help; have their friends help 'convince' them that they need to get help. Be careful though, you don't want to appear to have orchestrated this process by conspiring with others against them. That would be counterproductive.

A group of classmates were having a 40th class reunion at a meeting hall. They were having a great time catching up and sharing old stories and their current news. They noticed later however, that one of their formerly jovial and outgoing classmates was very subdued, quiet and reserved. One of them approached his wife and asked "So what's wrong with Bill, he is so different now?" The wife explained that he doesn't hear well and that he is embarrassed. She also mentioned that he actually brought hearing aids with him, but was embarrassed to wear them.

One of the female classmates took Bill aside and simply said "Why don't you go put on your aids and get back in the group. We don't care if you wear hearing aids, it doesn't bother us a bit. What does bother us is that we miss your big personality and funny humor. We miss YOU Bill!" He excused himself and went to another room, put in his hearing aids and came back to the party. Within a few minutes, he was starting to liven up, and by the end of the evening, he was as animated as ever, and he was so happy and grateful.

This story is extremely effective at illustrating why hearing is so important to us, and how effective hearing aids can really be. I have never heard of such a big turnaround in such a short amount of time. Bill went from glum wallflower to animated extrovert in the space of one evening.

This story is a powerful example of how someone can get part of their life back just by hearing others better. It simultaneously illustrates why getting over your own personal barriers is critical. As the story clearly reveals, the other classmates could care less about who wears hearing aids. It was an issue that Bill created in his own mind:

Fear of being seen wearing hearing aids matters less and less these days.

Summary

✓ The realization that there may be a problem can be painful.

✓ There are many reasons and excuses not to get hearing help.

✓ In a perfect world, people would just automatically get the help they need.

✓ Hearing loss is just another reminder of our advancing age.

✓ This is a medical condition; it doesn't fix itself and tends to get worse over time.

✓ There are many ways to help people get unstuck.

✓ Hearing loss can cause issues in and out of the home.

✓ In some cases, a hearing problem can be a safety issue.

Chapter 4

How We Hear

The human hearing system is an amazing sense that is central in our development from birth, and is what keeps us connected with others, all of our lives. When we are very small, it is our hearing that helps our brain figure out how to speak and say words. The fundamentals of speech itself are learned in part, through the ears. Facial expression and lip movement also help us decode what is being said to us.

When we are young, we hear the best that we ever will. Our young ears have the largest population of healthy nerve hair cells in our inner ear that they will ever have. Our middle ears have the best performance that they will ever have. And, our eardrums are the most sensitive that they may ever be.

Young people can hear sounds that even people in their mid-twenties may no longer be able to hear. They even have ring tones for their cell phones now that very few mid-twenty year olds or older can hear.

Hearing doesn't happen in the ears, hearing happens in the brain. While it is true that you cannot hear without ears, it is also true that sound means nothing unless the brain can interpret and understand its meaning.

Here is how it works

Sound waves of all pitches and from all angles and distances are funneled into the ear through the outer ear. The outer ear is naturally 'tuned' to the middle frequency of the human voice, but can also process a very wide spectrum of sounds easily. The sound waves are directed from the outer ear into the ear canal, and then to the eardrum.

The eardrum vibrates to the sound pressure of the sounds it is subject to and converts this sound pressure energy into a mechanical motion at the eardrum. The eardrum is the barrier that separates the outer ear from the middle ear. The eardrum is a three-ply membrane and is some of the thinnest skin in the body. It is paper thin; it is very strong and is very sensitive to sound.

The middle ear contains the smallest, most delicate bones in the body. The middle ear bones are the incus, malleus and stapes. In grade school they were referred to as the hammer, anvil and stirrup.

The job of the middle ear is to convert and amplify the vibrations from the eardrum and send this amplified sound to the inner ear that then converts the sound into electrical impulses, and sends these electrochemical impulses to the brain.

The Ear

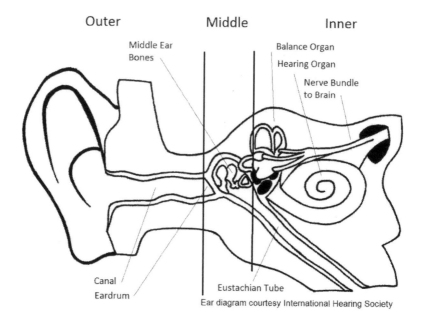

Outer   Middle   Inner

Middle Ear Bones

Balance Organ

Hearing Organ

Nerve Bundle to Brain

Canal

Eardrum

Eustachian Tube

Ear diagram courtesy International Hearing Society

Outer Ear - Funnels sound to the eardrum.
Middle Ear - Converts sound pressure to vibrations.
Inner Ear - Converts vibrations to nerve impulses.

With the two streams of information coming in from both ears, the brain combines the sounds to determine the meaning.

Having two ears is important for the following reasons:

- Stereophonic sound reception.

- Distance estimation of sound.

- Sound direction.

- Stimulating both sides of the brain with sound.

- Optimal auditory function.

- Provides better understanding in noisy environments.

Our highest pitch hearing fades after childhood

To illustrate how our hearing degrades from childhood into adulthood, consider the teenager loitering deterrent product called *The Mosquito*. This electronic sound amplifier dissuades teenagers from loitering in certain places. Teens loitering can tend to lead to crime and mischief.

Some audio engineers figured out that teenagers and young adults could hear high frequencies that mid-twenty year olds and older just couldn't hear. So, they produced a sound amplifier at a very high pitch that mostly only teenagers could hear.

What the teens hear is this horrible, mosquito-like high pitch sound, which is very uncomfortable. The sound is so annoying, that the teens will move out of range of it pretty quickly.

This technology has been used with great success and those people who were affected by the loitering reported a nearly 100% success rate. Teens and early twenty year olds would only hear a loud and blaring screeching sound that was simply intolerable after a minute or two, and they would be compelled to vacate the area.

More recently, teens can get ring tones for their cell phones in the range of hearing that their parents cannot hear. This idea has become wildly popular with them.

Hearing Happens in the Brain

Hearing doesn't happen in the ears, hearing happens in the brain. The ears collect and channel and convert sounds which become electrochemical impulses. The ears deliver two streams of information to the brain, which is continuously analyzing the sound stream for meaning and understanding.

Whether it is a speech sound, a machine sound, an animal sound or so on, our ears constantly take in and decipher the sounds around us. We are processing a wide variety of sounds that we sort through and classify, without even thinking about it.

Some sounds mean joy, some sounds mean danger and yet other sounds can be almost anything from useless noise, to extremely valuable information. We are constantly receiving sound stimuli and sorting them out for classification.

When we are listening to speech, the sounds of speech are broken down into phonemes and formants. These are the sound patterns of vowels, consonants, syllables and words that combine into sentences that we listen to, and then respond or react as we deem appropriate.

In the case of listening to music (without lyrics), we are not processing words, but we are processing sounds. The sounds of music, any music can be motivating or relaxing whether it is fast, slow, old or new.

All sounds, whether speech sounds, music sounds or any sounds, consist of frequencies and loudness. Frequency is also referred to as pitch. Low pitches are more bass sounding, while high pitch sounds are more treble sounding.

Human speech consists of combinations of low, medium and high pitches. Men's voices tend to be a lower pitch, and women's voices tend to be a higher pitch. This is because bigger vocal tracts make lower pitch sounds and smaller vocal tracts make higher pitch sounds. Men have larger vocal tracts than women, generally.

In musical instruments the difference between higher pitch sounds and lower pitch sounds versus size is this: An alto sax is a smaller saxophone and has a higher pitch sound. A baritone sax is a larger saxophone and has a lower pitch sound.

This gentleman in his mid-forties comes to me with his hearing problems, and his story. He is dating this gal with two young boys, and he gets along with them great. One day however, there is a tussle between the boys, and this guy hears what he thinks are bad words coming from one of the boys. He calls the boy out, and gets the mom involved, being concerned that this is a time to let the boy know that he shouldn't be speaking like that. As is turns out, he didn't quite hear correctly what the boy had said.

The boy was very emphatic to his mom and this guy about what he thought. There had apparently been other times when this gentleman's hearing wasn't the best, but this turned out to be the last straw. The boy told him: 'You either need to get a hearing aid, or break up with my mom.'

He was in my office within days, and his girlfriend's father bought him his hearing aids. He now relies on them every day, and comes right in if there are any problems. He knows that he isn't functioning nearly as well without his hearing aids.

You mean there is a clinical reason he can't hear me?

It can be true; he may hear his buddies just fine and not hear you very well at all.

There are two reasons for this: Women's voices are often higher pitch and have more vocal speech components than men: and, men's hearing loss is usually worse in the upper frequencies.

In some cases, a man can have a high pitch hearing loss and have normal hearing in the low pitches. If his buddies voices are lower pitched, he may have some trouble with their voices but can generally hear them okay. He will have the most trouble with women's and children's voices because they are higher pitched. Throw in a little background noise, and hearing can become very difficult.

Summary

✓ Hearing is vitally important.

✓ Our ears process a wide range of pitches from all kinds of sound sources.

✓ Our hearing is primarily designed for human speech.

✓ Our ears collect and process the sound, but we hear with our brain.

✓ Background noise makes hearing and understanding more difficult.

Chapter 5

Ignoring the Problem and Its Consequences

Your life won't end if you do nothing about your hearing problems. The process is usually so slow that it creeps into your life bit by bit. You get used to one limitation or another and that turns into the new normal. As time goes by, more and more things start getting added to the list. The TV has to be louder. You miss more punch lines. Understanding kids becomes difficult to impossible sometimes. You give up trying to carry on a conversation in a noisy place.

While some ill-effects of poor hearing may be annoying or embarrassing, they don't cause real harm. From a safety aspect however, a hearing problem can expose the sufferer to harm.

Here are a few safety concerns with hearing loss:

- Not hearing the knocks on the door that your house is on fire.
- Not hearing someone tell you watch out, that thing is going to hit you.
- Not hearing that car approaching.
- Failing to hear the crosswalk signal.
- Can't hear the train coming.

All of these things add up until finally, at some point or on some level, something has to give. There may come a 'pivotal moment' to provoke a change in thinking that can lead to at least seeking out a hearing evaluation. Or there is some incident that prompts a change which can lead to seeking help.

Other times, there may be no active action to address the issue, but rather, a path of avoidance is chosen, avoiding situations where hearing is an issue. Some people start to limit socialization that may include challenging listening situations. It is this avoidance path that robs the hearing impaired of the most quality of life. The long term and negative effects of avoidance can easily lead to loneliness, sadness and depression. All because of what usually amounts to a solvable problem.

Persons who already suffer from depression or loneliness can greatly amplify the effects of these issues with a hearing problem combined into the mix. Those with dementia or Alzheimer's and who suffer from hearing loss, can become much more anxious and paranoid when they cannot hear well in their already mixed up world. Hearing problems can compound and amplify other health issues.

Sometimes there can be an active reaction to hearing loss. Instead of avoidance, the hearing loss sufferer actively tries to dominate conversations by speaking and speaking, and not having to listen too much. This behavior of course doesn't promote balanced communication.

I was watching the news about a plane crash in Europe that had killed the Polish president and some of his staff. The story showed a video clip of people leaving objects at a makeshift memorial. One of the reporters said that people were leaving sandals at the memorial. I thought about this because I hadn't heard of this custom before. Sandals at a memorial? Okay. Seemed odd, but okay. Later I told my wife about the sandals at the memorial thing, and she looked at me kind of funny. I said that I hadn't heard of it either, but hey, they threw shoes at President Bush. Well, the story was repeated a day later, and both of us watched it. As it turned out, they weren't leaving sandals at the memorial, they were leaving candles. My wife gave me that look, and then simply commented: You should wear your hearing aids more often.

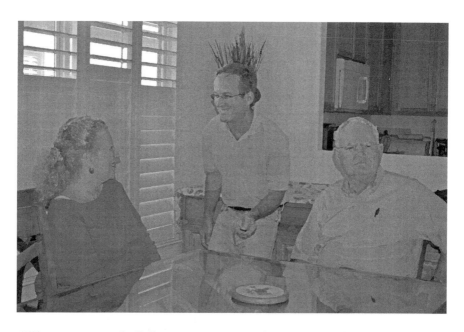

When you can't follow a conversation very well, you might as well be a million miles away.

There are clinical aspects to consider with an untreated hearing loss as well. Common nerve hearing loss over a long period of time can often result in neural atrophy. Basically, the nerves that send the signals from the ear to the brain tend to wither and diminish in their function if they are seldom or never used. It is very true that if you don't use it, you lose it.

When these nerves atrophy away enough, the listener's ability to understand words correctly begins to diminish. Left untreated, the hearing loss over a long period of time will leave the individual incapable of understanding speech very well, even with hearing aids.

So in short, it is easier for hearing professionals to help with a hearing problem if help is sought earlier. Waiting a long time to seek help can make it much harder to impossible to achieve success with hearing instruments.

Summary

✓ You can gradually become more and more disconnected from people and the sounds of life.

✓ Avoiding potential embarrassing situations can become a coping mechanism.

✓ Hearing loss can compound and amplify other health conditions.

✓ Waiting a long time to get hearing help can make hearing aids less effective.

Chapter 6

The Hearing Test

Person A   *Did you hear Joe passed away?*

Person B   *Oh, that's nice. (Not really hearing the message well)*

By the time a person is having trouble like the exchange above, they are probably, hopefully, starting to become aware that they may have a hearing problem. It doesn't take too many embarrassing or unpleasant misunderstandings to drive a person to sit in my chair for a hearing test.

Before going to the hearing test, consider taking your spouse or loved one, known in our business as the third party. Having someone there with you can help the hearing professional and yourself more fully understand your hearing problems and perhaps the problems caused by poor hearing.

Whether the third party is a spouse, child, sibling or even a friend or neighbor, if they are familiar with your problem, they can help.

Upon arrival at the hearing test office, you will be asked to provide some basic information, and most likely, take a survey to find out what hearing problems you are having. If someone familiar with your problem came with you, they may fill out a questionnaire about their experiences. This information helps the hearing professional assess your needs from a practical, everyday standpoint.

All of your information is protected per federal HIPAA privacy rules and guidelines. When followed properly, your information will be safeguarded at all times. If you apply for credit with a particular office, they may gather other information from you, and that information may not be protected under the same federal privacy rules.

You may be asked some beginning questions by the hearing professional like:

- What or who brings you to my office?

- Do you believe that you have a problem?

- How long have you noticed this problem?

- Do others notice a problem?

- Are other people commenting on your hearing?

Once the meet, greet, seat and the intake forms are done, the hearing professional will probably examine your ears, looking for:

- Any obvious sign of previous surgery

- Irregularities of the Outer Ear

- Amount and Consistency of Earwax

- Shape of the Canal

- Appearance of Eardrum

- Visible signs of Infection

- Foreign Objects

The hearing test itself will consist of any of the following:

Otoscopy - This isn't a test, but simply a look in your outer ear canal. Your ear canal should be free of excess wax, foreign objects, infection and generally be in good health.

Pure tone air conduction with inserts or headphones – This test is a set of tones (pitches) in each ear. There are low tones, medium tones and high tones. This is the heart of the hearing test and is one of the most revealing tests about how well you hear. This test is also the basis for setting up your hearing aid for programming by the computer.

Pure tone bone conduction – This uses your skull to send test tones directly to your inner ear. This test is to determine if there is a loss of hearing in your outer or middle ear.

Speech Reception Threshold – This is the level of speech loudness that you require to understand words.

Most Comfortable Speech Level – This is the sound level that you can easily understand speech at.

Uncomfortable Loudness Level – This is the loudness level of tones or speech that you find to be too loud for your comfort.

Word Discrimination Score – This test uses one-syllable words to measure how well you can decipher simple words. You are given a word at a level you can easily hear, and you have to accurately repeat it back. This is an important measure of how well you may or may not do with hearing aids.

Speech in Noise Test – As the name implies, this test uses increasing levels of speech mixed in with background noise, to determine how much noise it takes before you cannot understand the words very well.

Tympanometry – This is a measure of how rigid or flexible your ear drum is.

The Audiogram

The audiogram is a central element of the hearing test, whose results provide a 'picture' of how well you hear a series of tones in each ear.

Using the pure tone air conduction test, a range of tones is presented to each ear using headphones or foam ear inserts. The tones range from 250Hz to 8000Hz. What is revealed is what tones you can hear, and how soft or loud they need to be.

The results are plotted on the audiogram in graph format. At the top of the graph are the very soft sounds, and at the bottom of the graph are the very loud sounds. The left of the graph is the lowest tone or pitch (250Hz) and the right side of the graph is the highest tone or pitch (8000Hz).

The audiogram results are also a central component of programming hearing aids. The closer that the hearing aids are programmed to your needs, the better you will hear with them.

These marks are used to indicate your tone hearing test results:

Right = O

Left   = X

In the following simplified sample audiograms, you can see what marks equate to what hearing problems you may be encountering.

These are simplified examples, and are informational only. Your experience may be different. Note: Some offices test a very low tone of 125Hz.

A. Blank Audiogram

B. Legend Audiogram

C. Normal Hearing

D. Mild Hearing Loss

E. Moderate Hearing Loss

F. Severe Hearing Loss

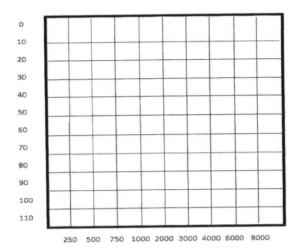

A. Blank Audiogram

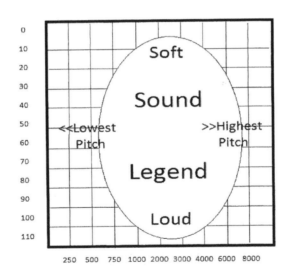

B. Sound Legend

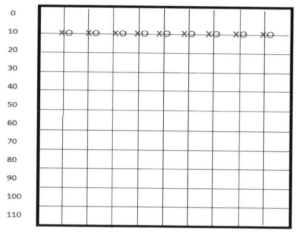

C. Normal Hearing (Hypothetical)

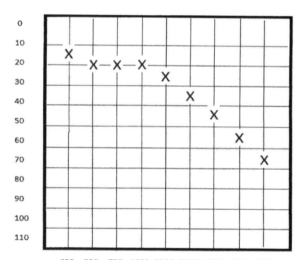

D. Mild Hearing Loss - Some difficulty in some situations (left ear shown)

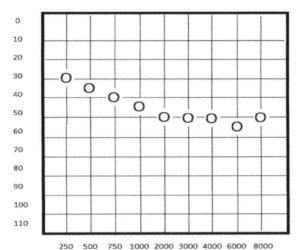

E. Moderate Hearing Loss - Difficulty in
many situations (right ear shown)

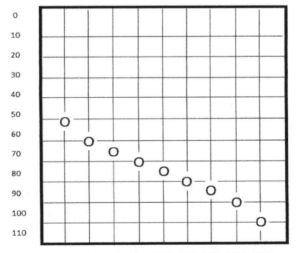

F. Severe Hearing Loss - Great difficulty
in every situation (right ear shown)

These tests all reveal something about how well you hear, and
how well you understand words, and what the overall health of

your hearing appears to be. These tests are valuable in answering questions like:

- Is there a problem with the hearing of tones?

- Are there any problems with speech recognition?

- Does some of the sound pass poorly through the middle ear?

- Is excess earwax to blame?

- Are there signs of disease or infection?

The hearing professional should explain the results of your testing, in terms that you can understand. It is the job of the hearing professional to give you an honest assessment of your hearing, and your options for getting help.

What I am looking for when I test you:

In my office, patients are evaluated from the moment we meet. I want to know:

- How loudly do I have to speak?

- Do I need to speak more slowly?

- How present of mind is the patient?

- What is their mood?

- What is their dexterity?

- Are there health issues?

- What led to the visit?

- What are their hearing test results?

- What if there is a hearing loss?

- Do they want help?

- Do they merit a medical referral?

- Will they need a medical clearance from an MD?

In some cases, there may be a test result that requires that you see your doctor about. Some examples of why you may need to see a doctor:

- Infection

- Foreign object in ear canal

- Injury to the ear

- Earwax

- Middle Ear problems

- Test results that may point to some other issue

In some cases, your doctor may be required to sign a medical clearance before you are permitted to purchase hearing aids. These laws vary by state and are in place to protect you.

In all cases, it is always in your best interest to talk with your doctor about your hearing if you know or suspect that you have a problem

Some Comments about Hearing Testing

You can go to ten different places, and have ten different experiences. Some places may test your hearing using eight tests and other places my only give you two tests. Some places will be concerned with how your hearing problems are affecting you and others, while other places may not care. Some places may want to pressure you into a purchase, others may not.

No matter what type of office you end up in to have your hearing tested, keep these basics in mind:

- Don't buy the first thing you see or listen to **unless** you really feel the provider is the one for you. Use your common sense.

- Talk to your friends and whomever you can about their hearing aids.

- Know your budget.

- Don't feel obligated to purchase instantly; it is a big decision.

- Check with your insurance, and VA, and state programs.

- Educate yourself; it is your hearing. Many online sites offer consumer analysis of products.

- If you trust the hearing professional, if they have a good reputation, and if the price doesn't seem excessive from what you know others are paying, then give them serious consideration.

After all of the hearing tests are completed, and there are no obstacles to proceeding, you will have a few choices:

- Do nothing (not a good choice).

- Get more testing?

- Shop Around.

- Purchase hearing aids.

Summary

✓ A comprehensive hearing test should include a number of tests.

✓ You should be evaluated not only with tones, but with words too.

✓ Your overall hearing health is being examined.

✓ Certain test results may require you to get a medical clearance from your doctor or other medical professional.

✓ Your test results should be explained to you.

✓ Your hearing aid options should be explained to you.

✓ **Bring a third party to the hearing test.**

Chapter 7

Buying Hearing Aids

"If I could have only one of my senses then I would choose hearing. Then I wouldn't feel so all alone." Helen Keller

Okay, so you are not deaf, but you are seriously thinking about possibly, maybe, perhaps buying hearing aids. Helen Keller's commentary on hearing leaves no doubt of her belief in the importance of hearing. She understood the importance and value of feeling like you belong and of being included.

You may not 'feel all alone' as she must have, but there is a reason why you are seeking help for your hearing. And more often than not, you end up in my office because of the influence of someone close. You are in effect, slowly becoming more and more alone, as you miss more and more around you.

Your problem becomes a problem for those who communicate the most with you.

The most common thing that many people in my office say is this:

'I can hear just fine.'

Trouble is that you don't know what you are missing. This is very important:

You won't miss what you never heard.

Statistics tell us that very few of the large pool of people who need help, actually seek it. For every six who could benefit from hearing aids, only one will seek help.

Take a look at a few of the negative ideas regarding hearing aids:

- Another part of me is failing.

- People will see that I have a hearing problem.

- It will make me look old.

- They are too expensive.

- I hate the stigma about them.

- I cannot justify the cost versus the problem.

- I don't trust hearing professionals.

- I can't stand feeling ripped off.

- I simply cannot afford them.

- I simply refuse to put up with wearing hearing aids.

Is it any wonder the number of hearing impaired people who seek to purchase hearing aids is so low?

These are all very valid reasons to put off and delay getting help. In fact, statistics show that the average person waits *five to ten years after noticing a problem,* to consider getting help and purchasing hearing aids. One could deduce then that perhaps the negatives and the stigma regarding hearing aids are the driving forces behind putting off getting help for a hearing problem.

If you find yourself beyond all of the barriers and obstructions to getting help, then you simply move on to the next steps:

- Finding a hearing professional

- Sorting through the dizzying array of choices in manufacturer and style of hearing aid.

Finding a Professional

The best advice for choosing a professional is to ask around. Talk to friends, loved ones, neighbors and whomever you can. Find out if they are happy or not. *If you find someone who likes their hearing professional, and is happy about wearing their hearing aids, then their professional may work for you also.*

In the hearing healthcare field, as with any other field, there are good practitioners, and then there are not so good practitioners. As a result, the hearing aid business sometimes has a less than wonderful reputation where the poor practices of a few can give the whole field a bad rap.

If you can't get a good referral from someone who is successful with their hearing aids, then you may want to consider some of these selection criteria:

- Clean office

- Friendly staff

- Friendly and knowledgeable provider

- Interested in why you are there

- Explains your problems

- Provides a hearing solution or range of solutions

- No excess pressure to purchase

- Reasonable prices

- Better Business Bureau recognized

In My Office

In my office, I meet all of the above criteria, *because it is what I would want if I were a patient.* You came to me for help, and I want to provide it, and I want it be a comfortable and informative experience. You may or may not decide to purchase, and this is okay. *What you will always walk away with is being better informed about your problem and your options.*

One of the very next things that I always do after the testing and the explaining is that I offer a demonstration walk with hearing aids on in my store. I work in a big box retailer, so I have two very different environments right inside the store. My office is a small, sound proof booth, and is very quiet. The store floor is more of a real world place, complete with background noise and plenty of auditory stimuli.

I take the hearing test audiogram that is in the computer, import it into a hearing aid software program, and I program the hearing aids for each ear's particular loss and at a beginner level. Once we have the sound not too loud and not too soft, the person is then sent for a walk around the store. There is nothing more powerful and convincing than to experience hearing aids first hand, in a real world setting.

Before the demonstration walk though, two important things take place:

I carefully set the levels of the hearing aids for the quiet office *and* the noisy store.

I carefully explain to the patient, that there is good news, and that there is bad news about wearing hearing aids:

The good news is that you can hear better.

The bad news is that you can hear better.

I make sure that they know and understand that they are going to start hearing things that they are not used to hearing. Some of these sounds will be useful; some of these sounds will be not so useful. It all goes together.

I program the hearing aids, based on the audiogram results and by applying my experience. I usually alter the initial settings for patient comfort and acceptance. Then, I fit the demonstration hearing aids into the patient's ears, and then I do something that nobody expects. I have the patient all hooked up with the hearing aids muted, so there is no sound yet.

Then I ask:

"How do they sound?"

It is amazing the variety of answers that I will get. They boil down to 'I can't tell the difference, and occasionally they will say, 'they sound great'. I then look at the patient and say okay, now let me turn them on.

I nearly always get a huge laugh from this little routine, and mostly from the third party observing, like the spouse. It is really funny as they watch me poke fun at the person in the chair. They get the joke, it is hugely funny, and it instantly reduces a lot of stress about the whole process.

Once the laughter dies down, and we enjoy the moment, then I level with the person, and we turn on the hearing aids.

The reasons for pulling this little trick are:

- It really eases the pressure.

- It adds a little humor to an otherwise somber process.

- It tells me if they can actually detect the difference in their hearing under amplification or not, or if they are just telling me what I want to hear.

Selecting a Hearing Aid

You can choose one or several places to get your hearing tested, and to see what the recommendation is. It is a good idea, though, to go into the meeting having an idea of what you may want. On the next page is a selection matrix to help narrow down your level of technology choices. Follow the instructions and see what outcome you get.

Selection Matrix Instructions

1. Read each statement in the matrix on the next page, and then circle the number under one of the three choices: Always, Some or Never. Do this for each statement.

2. At the bottom of the matrix, add the numbers from each column, from left to right.

3. Put the total from the columns in the grand total box

4. Compare this number to the legend following the matrix

Scoring: 7-10   Basic Technology

11-17   Mid-Level Technology

18-21   Best Technology

Selection Matrix

	Always	Some	Never
I go to meetings	3	2	1
I am still working	3	2	1
I have trouble hearing at home	3	2	1
I am in many different listening situations daily	3	2	1
I spend several days a week with children	3	2	1
I spend more than ten hours a week in public or in crowds	3	2	1
I go to loud places 2-3 times or more per week	3	2	1
Add the columns, then add the numbers in this row for grand total			
My total points >>>>>>>>>>>>>	Grand	Total >	

This is only a rough guideline and cannot take into account your particular circumstances. While I encourage my patients to buy the best that they can afford, I also tell some of them with the most severe hearing losses, that they may not really hear the difference from the most expensive models.

Basic Technology – These are simpler, more basic models with the least number of options and features and the least cost.

Mid-Technology – This group is the best choice for users who need something between basic and the best, which offers a few advanced features and mid-range pricing.

Best Technology – These are the best, most well optioned models with the latest features. These hearing aids have the best chance of adapting to a multitude of listening situations. They include the latest benefits from current research. They are also the most expensive.

Selecting a Style

Once getting your level of technology approximated, the next thing to decide is the style of instrument. You have several choices:

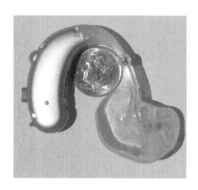

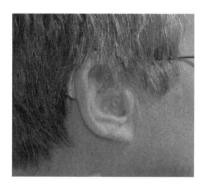

Behind the Ear (Power)   **Shown in ear**

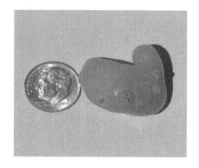

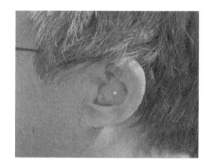

In the Ear   **Shown in ear**

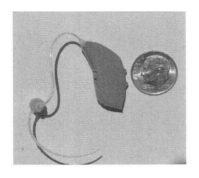
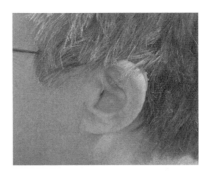

Thin Tube Behind the Ear   Shown in ear

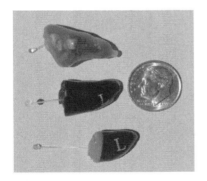
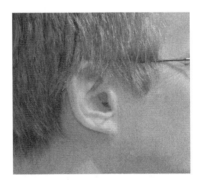

Completely in the Canal   Smallest one shown in ear

Completely In the Canal-These are almost invisible, and are not usually meant for more severe hearing losses

In the Ear-These hearing aids are visible without hair over the ears

Behind the Ear-This style includes small, open fit instruments all the way up to the largest power hearing aids, and are visible without hair over the ears. The much smaller, open fit hearing aid has become the most popular in recent years, due to the comfort and more natural sound. Its smaller size has also helped in its acceptance.

Your hearing professional will help guide you through the choices to arrive at a solution that makes sense for your lifestyle and needs. Some of my patients who are the most active need the best, most adaptable instrument, while others who don't get out much can get great utility from less sophisticated models.

In My Office

I always try to match the instrument to the person. I am looking for things like:

- How bad is the hearing loss?

- How powerful does the hearing aid need to be?

- What hearing aid configuration will best serve the patient?

- How can we hide it, or can we? Do they care?

- Can the patient deal with changing tiny batteries?

- Can they manage the controls and features?

All of these things are considered before I make my recommendation to the patient. We try to choose together what makes the most sense and what will serve them the best.

The time of selection is also the time when I make sure to counsel about proper expectations.

Hearing aids are not perfect, and they do not restore normal hearing.

Your voice will sound different to you, and you will probably hear more than you want to sometimes. Your hearing is not all better. All that we can do is work with your remaining hearing.

It is important to understand and accept that:

- Your old hearing is gone.

- Hearing aids will sound different.

- It will take time to get used to new hearing.

- There may need to be adjustments occasionally.

Why so expensive?

The pricing of hearing aids is all over the place. You can pay a fortune for one, and you can get one for less than the cost of a tank of gas for your car.

People always ask me, why is that little thing, that only amplifies sound, cost so much? I tell everyone that it isn't just the cost of the instruments themselves, but also the cost of the office and the staff to deliver and support these high tech devices.

You have to also consider, that teams of PhD's and Doctors of Audiology and engineers are designing and developing and continually improving hearing aids. This expertise drives up the cost for the latest, greatest things on the market.

One company was reported to have spent eight million dollars in R&D for their next family of hearing aids.

So you add up the fair cost of the hearing aids themselves, add in overheard of office, staff, taxes and some measure of profit, and you end up with some big numbers.

Big box retailers can offer significantly lower pricing, but they may not offer the nice big office and the same level of personal care that you may get from a smaller retailer.

Included in your purchase price is usually service after the fitting. This adds cost to support you after your purchase as well. Many retailers will offer 1-3 year warranty periods, during which time, all of your visits for service and adjustments are at no cost to you.

What should I buy?

You should buy what you can afford and will feel comfortable wearing. There are hearing aids that are so small now, that they are nearly invisible. Some of these types can make you feel all plugged up, but not all of them will. There are other hearing aids, called open fit, that go over the ear but are so small that just a little hair over the ears covers them neatly. The open fit is designed for mild to moderate hearing losses.

I like to fit the open ear models, because they are the most natural feeling that you forget that you have them on. The downside on this style is that past a certain level of hearing loss, the open fit style may start whistling when anything gets close to your ears.

For persons with a more severe hearing loss, we have to turn the hearing aid sound up quite a bit. When we turn the sound up, more sound wants to leak out of the ear, so we have to close the ear up by plugging sound from leaking out. When we do this though, it is called occlusion and it can make the hearing aid wearer feel plugged up; like they are in a barrel when they speak. The good news is that the increased sound levels can't leak out of the ear and back into the microphone, causing that high-pitch whistling that hearing aids can make.

For persons with a severe to profound hearing loss, we usually have to use a bigger, stronger in the ear hearing aid, or behind the ear model with a sound tube to deliver the sound to the ear.

Your hearing professional will help you narrow down your choices.

What should my hearing aids be set like?

Hearing aids can be set for fully automatic operation with no user controls, or they can come with a button to adjust to listening environments. Many can be ordered with a volume control. Fully automatic hearing aids are okay for some users, but they are not perfect for everyone. Volume controls are good for some users, but most people can do quite well with a push button. A push button allows you to change the mode that the hearing aid is in. Say for instance, Mode One is fine for quiet places, but is too loud in a noisy place. You can press the button on the hearing aid to Mode Two, and it will instantly be softer and kinder to your ears. Modes can be set up to match the acoustic environment that the wearer frequently encounters.

I set every one of my patients up for two modes of operation to match two key listening environments:

- Quiet Places

- Noisy Places

In quiet places you can have your best hearing and sound is turned up to your comfortable level. In noisy places, however, people are happier by turning sound down, especially the soft sounds, like background noise in public. Keep in mind though, hearing aids are not magic. We cannot help you get rid of all of the background noise.

Other modes that make sense can be:

- Noisier Places

- Music

- Assisted Listening (Public loop systems)

- Phone

- Blue Tooth

- MP3 Player

Note that some of these modes may require additional equipment to operate.

Internet Aids

There are a host of internet companies that will sell you hearing aids. You can test yourself on-line. You can dial in and get an adjustment to your hearing aid. You can do everything on the internet. This sounds like a great advantage and cost savings to many people.

The trouble is very, very few people possess the understanding and capability to accurately assess and then configure a hearing solution that makes any sense. There are simply too many variables and techniques that the average person cannot instantly master and the best website cannot figure out for you. Plus, the crucial in-store test-drive is not an option here

TV Advertised Sound Enhancers

If it sounds too good to be true, it probably is. Too many people tell me the same thing: I tried it and it didn't solve my hearing problems. Cheap sound amplifiers are just that: Cheap. They also broadly amplify all sounds, and only up to a certain range. People can very easily tell the difference between a highly engineered hearing aid, and a mass produced, low quality amplifier.

The bottom line is: Don't waste your money on TV sound amplifiers. There is no substitute for a well-researched and developed, precision hearing instrument, fitted properly by a competent professional.

Summary

- ✓ Very few with hearing loss seek help for it.

- ✓ There are many perceived negatives associated with hearing aids.

- ✓ Finding a professional takes due diligence on your part.

- ✓ You have to decide your quality and price range.

- ✓ Hearing aids need to be set for your comfort and benefit.

- ✓ Accept that hearing aids are not perfect.

- ✓ It will take time to adapt to hearing aids.

- ✓ Internet and TV hearing aids or sound enhancers are often disappointing.

Chapter 8

Life with Hearing Aids

When you leave the hearing office wearing hearing aids for the first time, expect some changes. I always tell my patients:

The good news is that I can help you hear better.

The bad news is that I can help you hear better.

You are now wearing high-tech programmable amplifiers that require regular care and maintenance. They change how you hear others, and they change how you hear yourself. So now you have these high-maintenance things that help you hear better, and you have this new hearing that requires plenty of time to adapt to.

When you are fit with hearing aids, we only give you about 65-70% of the sound you need, if you are new to hearing aids. As you get used them, we turn you up a little at a time. The acclimation time for hearing aids can be between 6-14 weeks. The best hearing aids today can turn themselves up over time, as you wear and acclimate to them.

In the beginning, you can wear them part time, or you can wear them full time. There are many different schools of thought about this. What I tell my patients is this: Wear them as much as you can tolerate in the beginning. You will do the best if you can get well acclimated early on with hearing aids.

I tell the patient that if the hearing aids are bugging them or if the sounds are just too much, turn them down or turn them off, or take them out and put them away and take a break.

Of course, if the hearing aids are too loud and bothersome, then I tell the patient that we should turn them down a bit. Every person perceives sound differently.

- Dialing in just the right amount of sound with hearing aids is very critical for patient success.
- People want to hear better, but they don't want to hear too much better.

You will spend the first few days wearing hearing aids just classifying sounds that are unfamiliar to you. Many times, patients comment on sounds that they have not heard for years-simple, ordinary sounds that most of us take for granted. So it truly is a good news/bad news thing.

Your own voice is the first thing that you will notice when you first start wearing hearing aids. You will hear yourself differently, just as you will hear others differently. Sometimes, you will hear yourself more differently than you do others. Other people's voices should be a bit louder and also clearer.

If your voice is too much different, then mention this to your hearing professional. Often times there are adjustments that can be made to soften the changes that hearing aids bring. Don't fall into the trap of thinking that your voice must sound exactly the same with or without hearing aids. If you are getting the amplification that you need, your voice will most likely sound different.

Having an open mind when you start wearing hearing aids is important. While they can help you hear better, not every listening situation will be ideal. Hearing aids cannot sort out the people you want to hear from those that you do not want to hear.

It is true that most hearing aids today can sort through speech and noise, but only to a limited degree. Aids cannot get rid of all the background sound, but they may help some.

Ideally, the hearing aid wearer will have some level of control over the hearing aids, in the form of a button, a wheel or in some cases, a remote control. When the wearer can change the loudness of the aids to match the surroundings, they can avoid getting 'blasted out' by too much sound.

I set my patients up for two modes if they are new to hearing aids: Mode or Program One is for Quiet Places and Mode or Program Two is for noisy places. In quiet places, we turn sound up to a comfortable level, and this setting is the best hearing mode. In noisy places, we turn sound down a little bit, especially soft sounds.

Hearing aids really need to strike an effective balance between their performance in quiet and their performance in noise to deliver maximum patient satisfaction.   Hearing well in a quiet home is nice, but being tortured with too much sound out of the home and in public can be a real problem for wearers.

The two most common complaints of new hearing aid wearers is background noise and sound quality. The hearing aids need to be set up to allow the wearer to be comfortable in a variety of listening situations.

For my patients new to hearing aids, they only get the two modes: Quiet Places and Noisy Places. Upon their follow up visit, we may adjust those modes a bit based on feedback the patient provides. We may also add a mode if they indicate a need that may be able to be addressed with another mode or function.

After they have been wearing hearing aids a while, then we may add another mode or functionality, based again, on patient feedback or needs.

Taking Care of Them

Hearing aids are a pain in the neck. There, now it is out in the open. It is true: hearing aids are expensive, they go in your ear, they can get clogged with wax, you can't get them soaking wet, you have to clean them, they need occasional adjustments, and on and on and on. They don't last much more than five to ten years and usually need replaced within 5-6 years. Some wearers get 10+ years out of them, but they are the rare exception, and not what is common. The two biggest reasons for getting new hearing aids is that they have a rough life, living in a difficult place-the ear. Secondly and perhaps most importantly is that advancements in hearing aids continually march forward. After a few years, you may be able to take advantage of a new or better feature that helps you even more than your old set of hearing aids.

When I am delivering and fitting the wearer for the first time, one of the things that I make sure I bring up is: Don't lay them around! I basically read them the riot act. If they are not in your ears, put them in their box or a protected place. Don't lay them on the coffee table; don't lay them on the end table. Don't lay them by the sink; don't leave them in the kitchen. Don't leave them loose in the car; don't put them in your pocket.

Take them off and put them in their box!

It isn't that hard. They are very easy to lose and they are pretty expensive things to just leave around.

So this gentleman is in my office telling me all about his poor experience at one of the national hearing chain stores. He tells me his sad story and then informs me that I am his last chance. These had better work, or he will throw them at me. Oh yes, he has a compressed time line and cannot wear them a full week before his follow up visit. No pressure.

The fitting comes, he is all set up, and I send him on his way for basically a weekend of use before a brief follow up, then a three week trip out of state. It is pretty much a make or break weekend for him and his new aids.

Well his next appointment was first thing Monday morning. Long about 9:56 or so, the customers started streaming in, and here he comes. He has this aggressively fast gait, and he has this intense look on his face. I am thinking to myself, he is either going to throw them at me, or kiss me.

He approaches me, both arms open wide, and he comes up and gives me a giant bear hug and exclaims: "These things are GREAT!" He was ecstatic with the performance with his new aids. His wife has stopped by my office several times thanking me. "You have no idea how you have improved our home life."

Well, I do know how I can improve your home life, I do it every day. And, my dad was my first patient while I was still training. Mom was probably the biggest benefactor of dad being able to hear much better. It was by her account, a godsend. Of course then, she didn't have to wear them.

Another thing that you have to do is to keep your hearing aids clean. Occasionally as needed, you need to wipe the wax away and clean off any lint or debris that may accumulate. It is a good practice to do this frequently. On some models, there may be a filter that needs to be changed. Your hearing professional will guide you in the care and maintenance of your hearing aids.

Earwax becomes an issue, too, when you wear hearing aids. Whether or not you have had trouble with wax in the past or not, if you produce wax and wear hearing aids, you may need to get on a regular cleaning schedule for your ears with your doctor or clinic. There are home cleaning kits available at many drug stores, but results can vary. Ears are not very easy to clean, so home cleaning kits may pose challenges for those with heavy wax.

Athletic things like sports and outdoor activities and workouts and so forth are an iffy arena for hearing aids. Some sports involve water and environments hostile to the hearing aids. Boating, for instance, is probably an activity for which you may wish to decide if you need your hearing aids or not. If you are the skipper, you may be least likely to fall overboard and most likely to need to know what is going on aboard your boat. Likewise, if you are a passenger and can hear okay enough to be safe, then perhaps the hearing aids should stay in their box and on shore.

Unlike glasses that can get wet and be dried off, hearing aids are not so lucky. If you get sprayed with a hose, it probably won't kill your hearing aids. If you have to dash from the parking lot to the car in the rain, it may not kill your hearing aids. If you get thrown in the pool, that may kill your hearing aids.

There are tiny microchips in each hearing aid, and water and moisture are not good for them. The moisture can start to cause corrosion which slowly eats away at the hearing aid circuits.

Moisture in the form of droplets can clog the microphone inputs and speaker outputs of hearing aids. The openings that collect sound and the openings that deliver sound are quite small. It doesn't take much of a drop of water or condensate to clog up a hearing aid.

Sweat is another thing that can literally eat your hearing aids. The salts and acids in our sweat are very bad for some hearing aids. The corrosive moisture can eat battery terminals in the course of a month. Luckily, manufacturers are getting better at moisture-proofing hearing aids, so this problem is much less of an issue today than it was 10-20 years ago.

Why do they whistle?

What we are doing when we amplify sound is basically putting sound into a hole that has a bottom. In the case of an ear, the bottom of the hole is the eardrum. As we put more and more sound in the ear canal (hole), there is more sound that wants to reflect back, or leak out of the ear. If too much sound reflects or leaks out, the excess sound gets back into the hearing aid microphone and causes that whistling sound associated with hearing aids.

There are two ways to reduce or eliminate feedback:

1. Decrease the gain of the pitch (frequency) of the hearing aid causing the feedback.

2. Keep more sound in the ear using standard-sized rubber tips or use inserts called ear molds, taken from an impression of your ear.

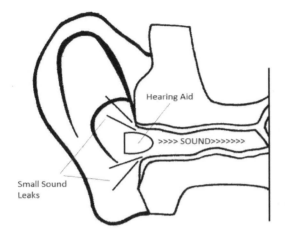

Hearing Aid with lower sound
input and little or no whistling

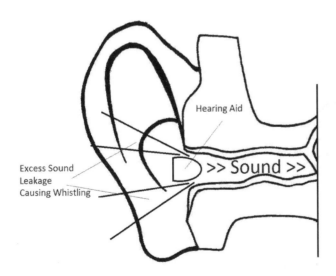

Hearing Aid with more sound in and excess
sound leakage causing whistling

Summary

✓ Better hearing can improve your home life.

✓ Expect your voice to sound different.

✓ It will take time to adjust to your hearing aids.

✓ Your hearing aids may need adjusted from time to time.

✓ New hearing aid wearers start out at a beginner sound level.

✓ You may hear sounds that you have not heard for a long time.

✓ Hearing aids require routine cleaning for best performance.

Chapter 9

Hearing Aids Don't Fix Everything

It is true; hearing aids cannot fix everything wrong with your hearing. In fact, all that we can do is make use of what remains of your hearing. There is no magic.

Sometimes people think that their spouse or loved one or friend who has purchased hearing aids is 'all better now'. I had one lady whose mom was fitted by another office, and they simply wanted them turned up. Turns out, the daughter wanted them turned up a lot. She actually went about 12 feet away and started whispering to her mom. At this point, I called time out and counseled the daughter on realistic expectations.

Realistic Expectations

It is very, very important in my work to make sure that I set realistic expectations for my patients. If I tell them the hearing aids will make them breakfast, and shine their shoes, they may be in for a letdown.

To tell people that the hearing aids will do more than maybe they can, may well lead to disappointment and possible rejection of amplification (hearing aids). You could take a perfectly good hearing aid fitting, and tell the patient it will be perfect, and when it isn't, they will be unhappy.

What you want to do is to take a good hearing aid fitting, and tell the wearer that it will help, but not be perfect. It will take time to adjust to, and things will sound differently at first. With realistic expectations and providing a solid fitting, the wearer has the best chance of success.

The best way to get the most from your hearing aids is to wear them, keep them clean and make sure that they are adjusted for your needs. Many times, we start you out with only 65-70% of the sound that you need. As you acclimate, we turn you up a little at a time. What this means is that you have to come see us once and a while.

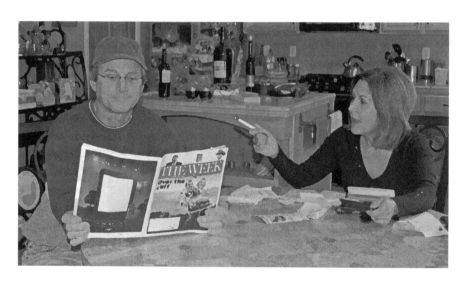

Hearing Aids can help him hear better, but they can't make him listen!

More sophisticated hearing aids have the ability to turn themselves up over time, as you wear them. This is handy as it reduces visits to the hearing office. Then again, visiting the hearing office once or twice a year isn't such a bad idea, especially if you start to have more difficulty hearing once you start wearing hearing aids.

Unlike the eyes, the hearing system cannot tolerate too much correction all at once. At the eye doctor, they can grind you lenses and you can see the best you can the same day. Not so with hearing aids. We start you out lower than your actual needs at first, then increase your sound levels as you get used to them. Each person is different, so there is no one rule for all people.

Modern hearing aids can store information in them about how you use them. This feature is often called data logging. Information is stored about how many hours the hearing aids are on, which modes you use, and what listening environments the aids are exposed to. Some hearing aids can help your hearing professional make settings changes to help you, based on the information from your hearing aid data.

The hearing aid can help provide clues if you are reporting a problem. Sometimes wearers don't fully understand how they are using their hearing aids. Say for instance, a patient comes in complaining about low sound. In most hearing aid models, you can view the data and figure out the problem. In this case, the wearer is turning the aids down unknowingly using one of the controls. This is very valuable data that helps us help you.

So a gentleman was in my sound booth office, and the door was open. Sitting just outside the door was his wife. I am in the booth with him, explaining to him some of the data that the hearing aids had collected. Well, he pretty much glazed over and was ready to fall asleep. I had his hearing aids out of his ears and on the computer. Since he couldn't hear very well at all, he bellowed out in a really loud voice: "Can it tell you how much sex that I have had?" I instantly turned bright red, and then looked out to see if his wife had heard this. Thankfully, she was oblivious to the comment. I went about my next tasks, quickly changing the subject. Later, I got up and closed the door. I sat down and leaned towards him, and I told him that the machine said that he had zero sex. He bellowed out "That's right!" And we both laughed heartily.

They think you are all better

Too often when someone starts wearing hearing aids, those around them think that their hearing is all better now. This isn't really the case. We can help you hear better, but we are working with what remains of your hearing.

The people you see most often may not realize that they may have some bad communication habits.

Here are a few examples of poor communication:

- Not in the same room.

- Too far away.

- Loud TV, radio or machine running.

- Not speaking face to face.

- Starting to speak face to face, then continuing to speak, while turning and moving away.

- Speaking too fast.

- Changing ideas too quickly.

- Dropping your voice as you continue to speak.

In My Office

I always counsel family members about many of the things outlined above. It really helps improve the odds of success for the wearer, if those around them have information and can do their part to promote the best communication. I tell the patient that they have done their part, now others have to help too.

Others can help in communicating with a person wearing hearing aids by keeping in mind all of the items noted above. Just a little bit of effort on everyone's part can produce in some homes, a much calmer and quieter place.

Summary

✓ Hearing aids don't make your hearing all better.

✓ As you acclimate, your sound level can be increased.

✓ Realistic expectations are vital to success.

✓ You may need a few adjustments from time to time.

✓ Family members can help by observing communication basics.

Chapter 10

Conclusion

Every so often, patients will respond to my suggestions of purchasing hearing aids, with something like "Why should I buy hearing aids if I am not going to live much longer?"

I come right back with "Because, in the first place, you don't know when your last breath is." Secondly, and most importantly, is the notion of why wouldn't you want your remaining time to be as good as it can be? Who wouldn't want this?

Yes, hearing aids are pricey and yet another thing to deal with and take care of, but getting part of your life back, in the sunset of your life can be priceless.

So often, first-time users in my office are a grandmother or grandfather who wants to hear their grandkids. They know that they are missing out on a richer relationship with the grandkids because of their inability to hear them very well. Young voices are some of the most challenging for people with a hearing loss to understand.

A story that really illustrates how poor hearing can rob you of your connections with others tells of this gal who decided to get a hearing test. At the intake, she mentioned she had quit one club, and was ready to quit another club or meeting, because of her poor hearing.

She did test to have a hearing loss, and I looked at her and said, "Don't you see? You are already becoming isolated from others because of your poor hearing. This is a shame, and it doesn't have to be like this." She was moved to act and purchased hearing aids.

It is like quitting smoking

It may seem very odd to compare success with hearing aids and quitting smoking.

Well, it is very simple:

The only people who are successful at quitting smoking are those who really *want* to quit.

It is the same with hearing aids; those who are successful with hearing aids are those people who really *want* to hear better.

Unrealistic Expectations

Too many people manufacture their own excuses and rationalizations to support their theory that hearing aids won't work for them.

The most popular method of proving that hearing aids won't work for you is to expect too much, and too often, way too much is expected.

Once your expectations haven't been met, boom! There you have it, proof positive that hearing aids won't work for *me*. This happens frequently in my practice. The perceived obstacles are made out to be insurmountable ones by the individual manufacturing unrealistic expectations which can never be met.

Popular Misconceptions

Too many people come to me with ideas and beliefs that are so totally false.

Here are a few:

- Hearing aids are all big, like geezers wear.

- Hearing aids will tell everyone that I am old.

- Hearing aids are really loud in noise.

- Hearing aids always whistle.

- Hearing aids can 'pick out' all sounds that I want.

- Hearing aids can block all sounds I don't want.

Misconceptions don't help matters when people are facing the prospect of purchasing hearing aids. When you combine high price, widely varying satisfaction, and the stigma many people associate with hearing aids, it is no wonder people use misconceptions as tools to prove that hearing aids won't help them.

Realistic Expectations, Reasonable Outcomes

Whenever I fit someone with a set of hearing aids, I make sure that they understand that:

- They are not perfect.

- There will be sounds that you want to hear.

- There will be sounds that you don't want to hear.

- Your own voice will sound different.

- Some listening situations will simply be difficult.

The Bottom Line

If you have a documented hearing loss, or even if others around you are telling you that you have a hearing problem, you owe it to yourself and others to at least check out hearing aids.

Get tested, and try them out. If they help, even just a marginal amount, your life can be better. If they simply don't work out for you, every place that you purchase from has anywhere from a 30-90 day trial period. You can return the hearing aids for a full refund for a limited time. In many states, it is state law that you must be allowed to return hearing aids in a specified time frame and receive all of you money back. Some states allow a restocking fee, which isn't refunded.

I have brought greater joy and happiness to many, many families by helping someone hear better. The large majority of people with hearing aids fitted properly are leading happier, fuller lives with less stress and anxiety.

What are you waiting for? Help yourself or someone you know get unstuck, and get the help that will make a difference.

Why on Earth would someone title a book 'Stick it in Your Ear'?

The title for this book comes from the usual response from people who are told or who suspect that they have a hearing loss. When told or reminded of a hearing problem, and hearing aids are suggested, most people's first reaction is something to the effect "Stick it in your ear, I won't even consider hearing aids".

Of course, if they do stick it in their ear, and it is an amplification device (hearing aid), they may be able to enjoy a greater quality of life. They can also bring greater peace to an entire household and circle of friends.

So, stick it in your ear really does encompass the entire spectrum or cycle that many people transition through, from early denial and non-acceptance, to actually sticking something in their ear to hear better, improving their life, and the lives of those around them.

And lastly, when I am teaching someone how to insert their hearing aids for the first time, I show them step by step how to do it. Then I hand the hearing aid to them and I tell them:

"Stick It In Your Ear".

ABOUT THE AUTHOR

The author is a licensed hearing professional who currently works at a big box retailer, selling and fitting hearing aids. It is a second career for him after a bumpy career in the tech industry. After a long period of unemployment, his family members were concerned about the future. Some suggested this, others suggested that. The father, with Alzheimer's disease, suggested hearing aids. As it turned out, the father was Patient Number One. The lessons of this first fitting were eye-opening and have led to a very successful practice improving lives every day.

5600524R00053

Made in the USA
San Bernardino, CA
13 November 2013